CONTENTS

The Small Steps. Big Rewards. GAME PLAN
is based on the lifestyle modification strategies
used in the Diabetes Prevention Program (DPP),
sponsored by the National Institutes of Health.
All of the DPP resources are available on the
Internet at www.bsc.gwu.edu/dpp/manuals.htmlvdoc.
This booklet may be reproduced without permission,
but should be acknowledged accordingly.

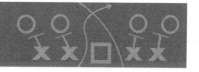

Diabetes prevention is proven, possible, and powerful.
Studies show that people at high risk for diabetes can prevent or delay the onset of the disease by losing 5 to 7 percent of their weight, if they are overweight—that's 10 to 14 pounds for a 200-pound person. **Two keys to success:**

• Get at least 30 minutes of moderate-intensity physical activity five days a week.

• Eat a variety of foods that are low in fat and reduce the number of calories you eat per day.*

In other words, **you don't have to knock yourself out to prevent diabetes.**

Have you wondered or possibly been told that you are at risk for developing diabetes or that you have pre-diabetes? To find out more about what things put you at risk, go to page 13 and read the "Are You At-Risk Check List" section. If you haven't already done so, be sure to talk with your health care team about your risk and whether you should be tested.

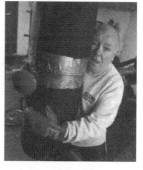

You don't have to knock yourself out to prevent diabetes. The key is: small steps that lead to big rewards.

* See Small Steps for Eating Healthy Foods starting on page 18 for examples of foods that are lower in fat and calories.

1

Small steps lead to big rewards.

When you take steps to prevent diabetes, you will also lower your risk for possible complications of diabetes such as heart disease, stroke, kidney disease, blindness, nerve damage, and other health problems. That's a big reward for you and your family and friends.

When you take steps to prevent diabetes, you will also lower your risk for possible complications. That's a big reward for you and your family and friends.

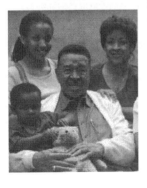

This ***Small Steps. Big Rewards. GAME PLAN*** kit is based on the Diabetes Prevention Program (DPP). This research study proved that type 2 diabetes could be prevented or delayed in persons with increased risk by losing a small amount of weight and getting 30 minutes of moderate-intensity physical activity, such as brisk walking, five days a week. We used the findings from the study to prepare this kit and to make it as easy as possible for you to take steps now to prevent diabetes. **Congratulations on taking your first small step!**

Here's what's in your GAME PLAN kit:

GAME PLAN Booklet—This booklet will help you take steps to prevent diabetes. Learn how to start your own GAME PLAN by setting goals, and tracking your progress. Learn more about pre-diabetes and your risk for getting diabetes.

Get healthy eating and physical activity tips to keep you focused and reach your goals. Learn more from the list of groups and websites that can help you lose weight and be more physically active.

GAME PLAN Food and Activity Tracker—This booklet will help you keep track of the foods you eat and how much physical activity you get. The DPP study showed that those who kept a daily log of their food intake and physical activity were more likely to lose the recommended amount of weight than those who did not. You can make more copies as you need them. Feel free to photocopy the Food and Activity Tracker pages at the back of this booklet.

GAME PLAN Fat and Calorie Counter—Use this booklet to look up the calories and fat grams in the foods you eat and drink and record the amounts in your Food and Activity Tracker.

Type 2 diabetes can be prevented ... by losing a small amount of weight and getting 30 minutes of activity, such as brisk walking, five days a week.

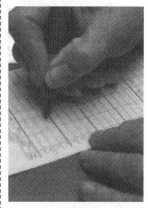

Those who kept a daily log of food intake were more likely to lose the recommended amount of weight than those who did not.

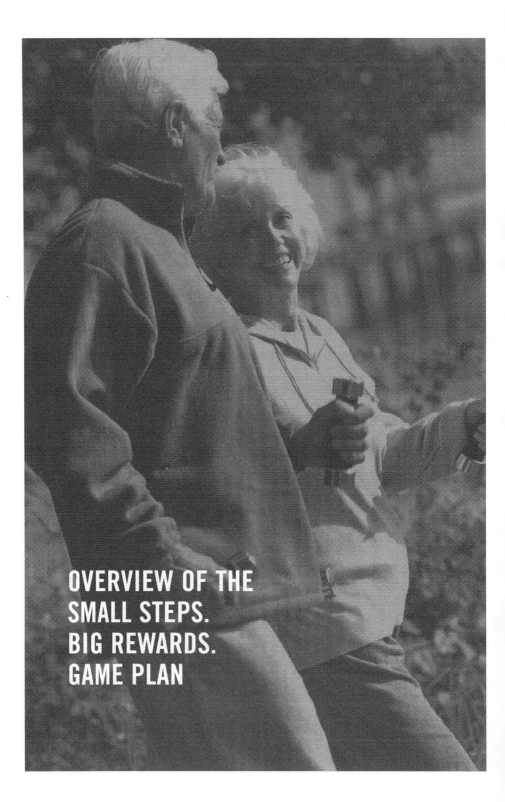

OVERVIEW OF THE
SMALL STEPS.
BIG REWARDS.
GAME PLAN

One Small Step: *Know your risk.* Work with your health care team to find out if you have pre-diabetes, a condition that puts you at risk for type 2 diabetes. Learn more about your risk for diabetes on page 13.

Big Reward: Knowing you can prevent or delay diabetes can give you peace of mind. Ask yourself these questions and write down your answers.

Why do you want to prevent diabetes?_____

_____

_____

Who do you want to do it for?_____

_____

_____

Review your answers every week to help you stay with your GAME PLAN.

One Small Step: *Start your GAME PLAN.* Use this booklet to create your own GAME PLAN to prevent diabetes. Work with your health care team, family, and friends. All of you can form a winning team to prevent diabetes. Here's how to get started.

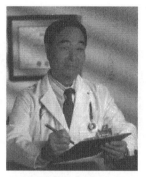

Find out if you are at risk for diabetes. Talk to your health care provider.

Plan to set a weight loss goal: The key to preventing diabetes is to lose weight by eating healthy foods that are lower in fat and calories and being physically active. Set a goal that you can achieve. A good goal is to lose at least 5 to 10 percent (10 to 20 pounds if you weigh 200 pounds) of your current weight. A 5 to 7 percent weight loss was shown to have a big impact on lowering the risk of diabetes in the DPP study.

Here's how to figure out your weight loss goal. Multiply your weight by the percent you want to lose. For example, if John weighs 240 pounds and wants to lose 7 percent of his weight, he would multiply 240 by .07.

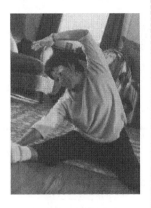

Losing 5 to 7 percent of your weight is one big step to reduce your risk of diabetes.

240 pounds	240 pounds
x .07 (7 percent)	- 17 pounds
16.8 pounds	223 pounds

John's goal is to lose about 17 pounds and bring his weight down to 223 pounds.

Choose your weight loss goal:
My 5 percent goal will be to lose _____ pounds.
My 7 percent goal will be to lose _____ pounds.
My 10 percent goal will be to lose _____ pounds.

Now, start thinking about how much better you will feel when you reach your goal. Keep in mind that losing even a small amount of weight can help you prevent diabetes. Weigh yourself at least once a week and write down your progress. Research shows that people who keep track of their weight reach their goals more often than those who don't.

Eat healthy foods: Make healthy food choices to help reach your weight loss goal. There are many weight loss plans from which to choose. But the DPP showed that you can prevent or delay the onset of diabetes by losing weight through a low-fat, reduced calorie eating plan, and by increasing physical activity. Use the tips on pages 18–25 to eat healthy and help you reach your goals.

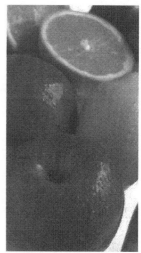

Make healthy food choices to help reach your weight loss goal.

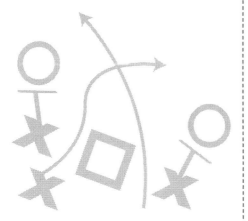

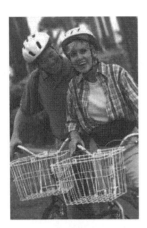

Try dancing, swimming, biking, walking, or any activity that keeps you moving for 30 minutes most days.

Figure out how many calories and fat grams you should have per day. Use this chart to figure out your goals for losing one to two pounds per week.

Recommended Calories and Fat Grams Daily
**It is not advised to eat less than 1,200 calories a day

Current Weight	Calories and Fat Grams per day
120 –170 pounds	1,200 calories a day 33 grams fat a day
175 – 215 pounds	1,500 calories a day 42 grams fat a day
220 – 245 pounds	1,800 calories a day 50 grams fat a day
250 – 300 pounds	2000 calories a day 55 grams fat a day

Source: DPP Lifestyle Manual of Operations

My goal is to eat no more than _____ calories and _____ grams of fat per day. Use the Fat and Calorie Counter to help you keep track of the number of fat grams and calories you take in each day.

Move more: When you move more every day, you will burn more calories. This will help you reach your weight loss goal. Try to get at least 30 minutes of moderate-intensity physical activity five days a week. If you have not been active, start off slowly, building up to your goal. Try brisk walking, dancing, swimming, biking, jogging, or any physical activity that helps get your heart rate up. You don't have to get all your physical activity at one time. Try getting some physical activity throughout the day in 10 minute sessions. Use the tips on pages 28-33 to get moving toward your goals.

My goal is to start out by getting at least _____ minutes of physical activity _____ days per week and to build up to 30 minutes, five days a week.

Big Reward: Losing weight by eating healthy and getting more physical activity not only can help you prevent diabetes, but it also lowers your risk for heart disease, certain types of cancer, arthritis, and many other health problems. Also, you will feel better, and have more energy to do the things you enjoy.

One Small Step: *Track your GAME PLAN progress.* Write down your goals in the GAME PLAN Food and Activity Tracker. Make copies of the tracker and keep them with you. Write down everything you eat and drink. Then, when you have time, use the GAME PLAN Fat and Calorie Counter booklet to add up your calories and fat grams for the day.

Big Reward: Keeping track of what you eat and drink and how many minutes of physical activity you get each day is one of the best ways to stay focused and reach your goals. As you lose weight, you will feel better about yourself and about reaching your goal.

It is important to find out early if you have diabetes or if you are at risk for developing it.

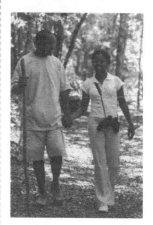

9

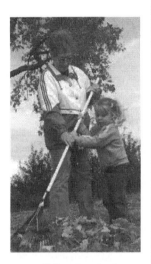

Take your next small step now! Add one or two healthy changes every week.

One Small Step: *Start your own team to prevent diabetes.* You don't have to prevent diabetes alone. Invite other people to get involved. Try teaming up with a friend or family member. Start a local walking group with your neighbors or at work or at your church. Trade healthy recipes and weight loss tips with your co-workers. Tell other people about the small steps you are taking to prevent diabetes and make sure you help each other stick to your GAME PLANs.

Big Reward: When you involve other people in your GAME PLAN, you will be more likely to stay at it and you will be helping others to prevent diabetes and other health problems.

Take your next small step now! Add one or two healthy changes every week. If you fall off the wagon, don't get down on yourself. Review your GAME PLAN and get back on track. It's not easy to make lifelong changes in what you eat and in your level of physical activity, but you can use the tips and ideas in this booklet to help you stick to your goals and succeed. And remember: **Preventing diabetes is good for you and for your family and friends. Keep at it!**

AM I AT RISK FOR
TYPE 2 DIABETES
AND PRE-DIABETES?

What is diabetes?

Almost 21 million Americans have diabetes, a serious disease in which blood glucose (blood sugar) levels are above normal. Most people with diabetes have type 2, which used to be called adult-onset diabetes. At one time, type 2 diabetes was more common in people over age 45. But now more young people, even children, have the disease because many are overweight or obese.

At least 54 million Americans have pre-diabetes and are more likely to go on to develop diabetes within 10 years.

Diabetes can lead to problems such as heart disease, stroke, vision loss, kidney disease, and nerve damage. About one-third of people with type 2 diabetes do not even know they have it. Many people do not find out they have diabetes until they are faced with problems such as blurry vision or heart trouble. That's why you need to know if you are at risk for diabetes.

What is pre-diabetes?

At least 54 million Americans over age 20 have pre-diabetes. Before people develop type 2 diabetes, they usually have "pre-diabetes"—that means their blood glucose levels are higher than normal, but not yet high enough to be called diabetes. People with pre-diabetes are more likely to develop diabetes within 10 years and they are more likely to have a heart attack or stroke.

12

Are You At-Risk Check List

Find out if you are at risk for diabetes and pre-diabetes.

There are many factors that increase your risk for diabetes. To find out about your risk, check each item that applies to you.

❏ I am 45 years of age or older.

❏ The At-Risk Weight Chart on page 15 that shows my current weight puts me at risk.

❏ I have a parent, brother, or sister with diabetes.

❏ My family background is African American, Hispanic/Latino, American Indian, Asian American, or Pacific Islander.

❏ I have had diabetes while I was pregnant (this is called gestational diabetes) or I gave birth to a baby weighing 9 pounds or more.

❏ I have been told that my glucose levels are higher than normal.

❏ My blood pressure is 140/90 or higher, or I have been told that I have high blood pressure.

❏ My cholesterol (lipid) levels are not normal. My HDL cholesterol ("good" cholesterol) is less than 35 or my triglyceride level is higher than 250.

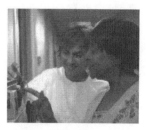

Almost 21 million Americans have diabetes— one-third don't even know it. You need to know if you are at risk for diabetes.

❑ I am fairly inactive. I am physically active less than three times a week.

❑ I have been told that I have polycystic ovary syndrome (PCOS).

❑ The skin around my neck or in my armpits appears dirty no matter how much I scrub it. The skin appears dark, thick and velvety. This is called acanthosis nigricans (A-can-THO-sis NI-gri-cans).

❑ I have been told that I have blood vessel problems affecting my heart, brain, or legs.

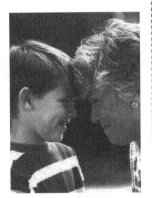

There are many factors that increase your risk for diabetes.

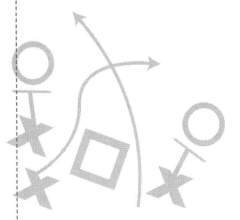

AT-RISK WEIGHT CHARTS

Find your height in the correct chart. If your weight is equal to or greater than the weight listed, you are at increased risk for type 2 diabetes.

IF YOU ARE NOT ASIAN AMERICAN OR PACIFIC ISLANDER AT RISK BMI ≥ 25		IF YOU ARE ASIAN AMERICAN AT RISK BMI ≥ 23		IF YOU ARE PACIFIC ISLANDER AT RISK BMI ≥ 26	
HEIGHT	WEIGHT	HEIGHT	WEIGHT	HEIGHT	WEIGHT
4'10"	119	4'10"	110	4'10"	124
4'11"	124	4'11"	114	4'11"	128
5'0"	128	5'0"	118	5'0"	133
5'1"	132	5'1"	122	5'1"	137
5'2"	136	5'2"	126	5'2"	142
5'3"	141	5'3"	130	5'3"	146
5'4"	145	5'4"	134	5'4"	151
5'5"	150	5'5"	138	5'5"	156
5'6"	155	5'6"	142	5'6"	161
5'7"	159	5'7"	146	5'7"	166
5'8"	164	5'8"	151	5'8"	171
5'9"	169	5'9"	155	5'9"	176
5'10"	174	5'10"	160	5'10"	181
5'11"	179	5'11"	165	5'11"	186
6'0"	184	6'0"	169	6'0"	191
6'1"	189	6'1"	174	6'1"	197
6'2"	194	6'2"	179	6'2"	202
6'3"	200	6'3"	184	6'3"	208
6'4"	205	6'4"	189	6'4"	213

Source: *Adapted from Clinical Guidelines on the Identification, Evaluation, and Treatment of Overweight and Obesity in Adults: The Evidence Report*

What is the next step?

If you have checked any of the items on pages 13 or 14, be sure to talk to your health care team about your risk for diabetes and whether you should be tested.

- If you are age 45 or older, testing for pre-diabetes and diabetes should be considered, especially if you have an at-risk weight according to the charts on page 15.

- If you are age 45 or older without any risk factors, ask about your risk for pre-diabetes or diabetes and if you should get tested.

- If you are 20 to 44 years old, have an at-risk weight, and have checked any other items on pages 13 or 14, ask about your risk for pre-diabetes or diabetes and if you should get tested.

- Repeat testing should be done every 3 years.

Be sure to talk to your health care team about your risk for diabetes and whether you should be tested.

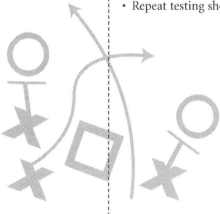

Know Your Blood Glucose Numbers

	Fasting Blood Glucose Test	2-Hour Oral Glucose Tolerance Test
Normal	Below 100	Below 140
Pre-diabetes	100 - 125	140 - 199
Diabetes	126 or above	200 or above

Ask your health care team about these tests and ask for your blood glucose numbers. It is important to find out early if you have pre-diabetes or type 2 diabetes, because early treatment can prevent the serious problems caused by high blood glucose.

Medicare Benefits for People At Risk for Diabetes

For people with Medicare who are at risk for diabetes, Medicare covers a screening blood glucose test to check for diabetes. If you are obese or have a history of high blood glucose, high blood pressure, high cholesterol, or other risk factors, you may qualify for this test. Based on the test results, you may be able to get up to two screening tests per year. Medicare covers the full cost of this screening test. For more information, go to: www.medicare.gov/health/diabetes.asp.

Type 2 diabetes is a serious disease but it can be prevented or delayed. Take steps now to lower your risk for diabetes.

It is important to find out early if you have pre-diabetes or type 2 diabetes, because early treatment can prevent the serious problems caused by high blood glucose.

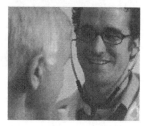

SMALL STEPS
FOR EATING
HEALTHY FOODS

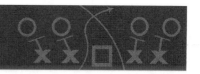
When it comes to eating healthy to lose weight, the three most important steps are:

1. Take in fewer calories than you burn during the day.

2. Eat less fat (especially saturated fats and trans fats—see page 20) than you currently eat.

3. Eat smaller portions of high fat and high calorie foods than you currently eat.

Portion sizes are often smaller than we think. Use this chart as a guide for portion sizes:

	Portion Size	*Same size as*
	1/2 cup of cooked rice or pasta	An ice cream scoop
	1 1/2 ounces of low-fat cheese	Four dice
	3 ounces of lean meat or fish	A deck of cards or a cassette tape
	2 tablespoons low-fat peanut butter	A ping pong ball

19

Use the Fat and Calorie Counter to look up the number of grams of fat and the number of calories in the foods you eat.

Remember: The key to losing weight and preventing diabetes is to make lifelong changes—not quick fixes—that work for you. While some diets may be popular now, there is no proof about their long-term success or if they can prevent diabetes. But the DPP showed that you can prevent or delay the onset of diabetes by losing weight through a low-fat, reduced calorie eating plan, and by increasing physical activity.

Saturated fat is found mostly in foods that come from animals like fatty cuts of beef, lamb, pork, poultry with skin, whole and 2% milk, butter, cheese, and lard. It can also be found in palm and coconut oil.

Trans fat is found in some of the same foods as saturated fat, such as vegetable shortening and hard or stick margarine. It can also be found in processed foods that are made with partially hydrogenated vegetable oils, for example, cookies, baked goods, fried foods and salad dressings.

The key to losing weight and preventing diabetes is to make lifelong changes—not quick fixes—that work for you.

Eat a Variety of Healthy Foods From Each Food Group

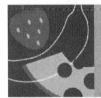

Focus on fruits. Eat a variety of fruits—whether fresh, frozen, canned, or dried—rather than fruit juice for most of your fruit choices. For a 2,000-calorie diet, you will need 2 cups of fruit each day (for example, 1 small banana, 1 large orange, and 1/4 cup of dried apricots or peaches).

Vary your veggies. Eat more dark green veggies, such as broccoli, kale, and other dark leafy greens; orange veggies, such as carrots, sweetpotatoes, pumpkin, and winter squash; and beans and peas, such as pinto beans, kidney beans, black beans, garbanzo beans, split peas, and lentils.

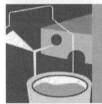

Get your calcium-rich foods. Get 3 cups of lowfat or fat-free milk—or an equivalent amount of low-fat yogurt and/or low-fat cheese (11/2 ounces of cheese equals 1 cup of milk)—every day. For kids aged 2 to 8, it's 2 cups of milk. If you don't or can't consume milk, choose lactose-free milk products and/or calcium-fortified foods and beverages.

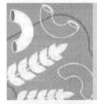

Make half your grains whole. Eat at least 3 ounces of whole-grain cereals, breads, crackers, rice, or pasta every day. One ounce is about 1 slice of bread, 1 cup of breakfast cereal, or 1/2 cup of cooked rice or pasta. Look to see that grains such as wheat, rice, oats, or corn are referred to as "whole" in the list of ingredients.

Go lean with protein. Choose lean meats and poultry. Bake it, broil it, or grill it. And vary your protein choices—with more fish, beans, peas, nuts, and seeds.

Know the limits on fats, salt, and sugars. Read the Nutrition Facts label on foods. Look for foods low in saturated fats and trans fats. Choose and prepare foods and beverages with little salt (sodium) and/or added sugars (caloric sweeteners).

Take these small steps to eat healthy:

A healthy eating plan is one that:

- Highlights eating fruits, vegetables, whole grains, and fat-free or low-fat milk, and milk products.
- Includes lean meats, poultry, fish, beans, eggs, and nuts.
- Is low in saturated fats, *trans* fats, cholesterol, salt (sodium), and added sugars.

Keep these healthy eating tips in mind:

- Try not to exceed the amount of calories and fat grams that you need on a daily basis.
- Try to eat meals and snacks at regular times every day.
- Make less food look like more by serving your meals on a smaller plate.
- Take your time when you eat. It takes about 20 minutes for your stomach to tell your brain that you are full.
- Try to limit your alcoholic beverage intake. If you drink alcohol, chose light beer and avoid mixed drinks.

At home:

- Choose foods that are not fried. Instead of fried chicken, try it grilled or baked. Instead of greasy french fries or potato chips, slice potatoes, mix them with a little bit of oil, herbs, and pepper, and bake them in the oven.
- Lighten your recipes by using reduced-fat (light) or fat-free versions of items such as sour cream,

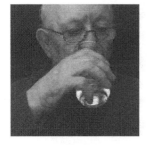

Drink lots of water.

cream cheese, mayonnaise, cheese and salad dressing.

- Use herbs and seasonings to add flavor to low-fat dishes. Instead of salt, give foods a little kick by adding hot sauce or red pepper flakes.
- Wrap up and refrigerate leftover foods right after cooking so you're less tempted to go back for seconds.
- Make time to cook healthy main dishes, casseroles, or soups. Freeze portions so you have healthy meals ready for days when you are too busy or too tired to cook.
- For dessert, eat a piece of fruit. Also, try fat-free or low-fat frozen yogurt or sherbet instead of ice cream. Instead of cakes or brownies, have one scoop of vanilla fat-free frozen yogurt with a tablespoon of fat-free chocolate sauce on top.

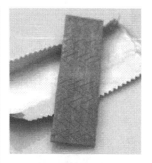

Chew sugar-free gum between meals to help cut down on snacking.

In-between meals:
- Replace snacks high in fat with crunchy fruits, vegetables, or a tablespoon or two of unsalted nuts.
- Drink lots of water. Choose water or sugar-free soda instead of a regular 20-ounce soda or juice drink. By doing this, you can cut about 250 calories.
- Chew sugar-free gum between meals to help cut down on snacking. Reach for a piece of gum or a hard candy instead of a snack high in fat or calories.

23

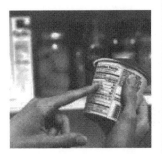

Read and compare food labels when shopping.

When shopping:

- Make a list of what you need ahead of time and try to stick to it.
- Avoid going shopping when you are hungry. Often, you will end up with things you really don't want or need.
- Read and compare food labels when shopping. Choose foods with fewer calories and that are lower in saturated fats, trans fats, cholesterol and sodium. Check the serving size and the number of servings in the package on the label.
- Buy a variety of fruits, vegetables, and whole grain foods. Try a new fruit or vegetable each week, such as kiwi fruit or butternut squash.
- Choose reduced-fat or light versions of mayonnaise, cheese, and salad dressing. Use fat-free or 1 percent low-fat milk instead of whole milk.
- You know best what high-calorie foods tempt you the most, such as cookies, cake, ice cream and snacks. Make it easy on yourself: Don't have them in your home, your office, or anywhere else.

At work or on the run:

- Bring your lunch to work so you can take charge of what you eat. Make a sandwich with whole grain bread and turkey or lean beef. Use mustard or a little bit of "light" mayonnaise. Pack carrots and celery sticks instead of chips. Choose low-fat/fat-free milk, water, or other drinks without added sugar.
- Pack a healthy snack in case you get hungry. Try an apple, a banana, a cup of fat-free yogurt, or reduced-fat or light string cheese sticks.
- Try to pack your lunch the night before so it's ready to go when you are.
- Take a different route to work to avoid passing by tempting high-calorie foods at nearby restaurants, bakeries, or stores.

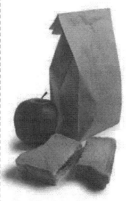

Bring your lunch to work so you can take charge of what you eat.

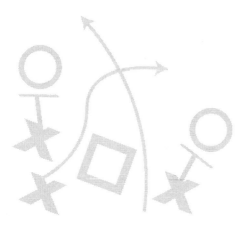

When eating out:

- Take time to look over the menu and make a healthy choice.
- Don't be afraid to ask for items not on the menu or to have a meal prepared with less or no added fat.
- Ask about portion sizes and the fat and calorie content of menu items.
- Choose steamed, grilled, or broiled dishes instead of those that are fried or sautéed.
- Be the first to order so you are not influenced by what others are ordering.
- Always order the smallest size meal instead of the larger, super-sized versions at fast-food restaurants.
- You can eat half of what you order and take the rest home for a second meal.
- Order salad dressing, gravy, sauces, or spreads "on the side."
- Order a salad for starters and share a main dish with a friend.
- When you crave high-calorie foods, desserts, or snacks, don't be too hard on yourself. It's okay to have a small portion once in a while or to share a dessert with a friend. Just keep your weight loss goal in mind.
- Stay away from "all-you-can-eat restaurants or buffets" where it's hard to control portion sizes and how much you eat.

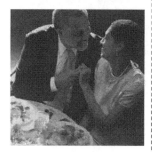

Take time to look over the menu and make a healthy choice.

These healthy eating tips are examples of the small steps you can take to jumpstart your GAME PLAN. Try a few new steps each week. Once you get going, you'll find lots of other ways to make small changes.

For more ideas and help, check your local library or bookstore for healthy cookbooks and weight loss books. These web sites have lots of ideas as well.

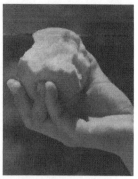

Once you get going, you'll find lots of other ways to make small changes.

United States Department of Agriculture (USDA)
www.nutrition.gov

Dietary Guidelines for Americans
www.healthierus.gov/dietaryguidelines

Food and Drug Administration's (FDA) Nutrition Facts Label
www.cfsan.fda.gov/~dms/foodlab.html

My Pyramid: Steps to a Healthier You
www.MyPyramid.gov

National Heart, Lung, and Blood Institute
www.nhlbi.nih.gov

Weight-Control Information Network
www.win.nih.gov/index.htm

American Diabetes Association
www.diabetes.org

American Dietetic Association
www.eatright.org

27

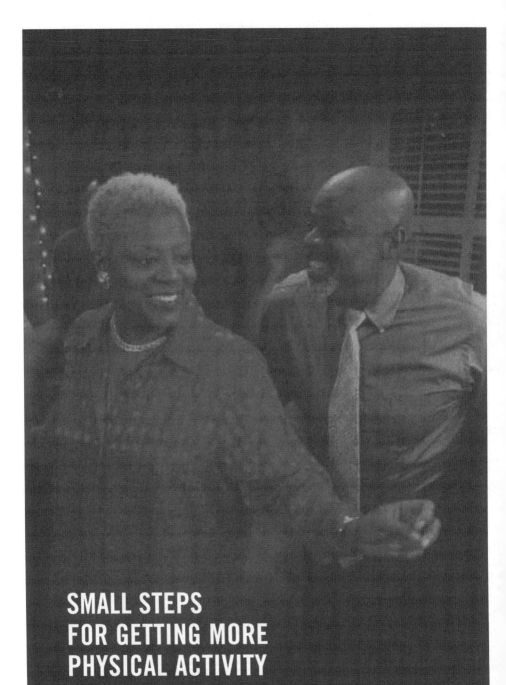

**SMALL STEPS
FOR GETTING MORE
PHYSICAL ACTIVITY**

The Diabetes Prevention Program (DPP) showed that you could prevent or delay the onset of diabetes by losing weight through small changes in eating and physical activity. To help lose weight, most of the people in the study who made lifestyle changes chose walking briskly for 30 minutes, 5 days a week.

There are lots of things you can do at home and at work to get more physical activity throughout the day. You don't have to play a sport or go to a gym to be more active, unless that's what you like to do. You can walk or try swimming, water aerobics, biking, dancing, or any activity that keeps you moving toward the goal of 30 minutes of moderate-intensity physical activity five days a week. Before you start a physical activity program, be sure to talk with your health care provider.

Use these tips to get started, keep you moving, and make your physical activity time more fun.

You don't have to play a sport or go to a gym to be more active, unless that's what you like to do.

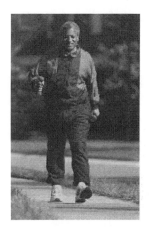

Dress to move. Wear supportive shoes with thick, flexible soles that will cushion your feet and absorb shock.

Dress to move.

Wear supportive shoes with thick, flexible soles that will cushion your feet and absorb shock. Your clothes should allow you to move, and keep you dry and comfortable. Look for synthetic fabrics that absorb sweat and remove it from your skin.

Start off slowly.

Start off by taking a 5-minute walk (or doing another physical activity that you like) on most days of the week. Slowly, add more time until you reach at least 30 minutes of moderate-intensity physical activity five days a week.

Build physical activity into your day.

Start or end your day by taking your dog—or a friend's dog—for a brisk walk. When shopping, park a little further away from the store's entrance. If it's safe, get off the bus a stop or two before your work place and walk the rest of the way. While watching TV, walk or dance around the room, march in place, or do some sit-ups and leg lifts. Double bonus: cut out a TV show and get moving instead!

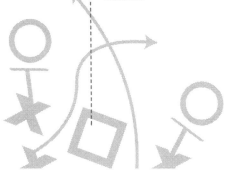

Move more at work.

Try to get a "movement break" during the day. Take a walk during lunchtime. Deliver a message in person to a coworker instead of sending an email. Walk around your office while talking on the telephone. Take the stairs instead of the elevator to your office.

Count your steps.

You may be surprised to learn how much walking you already do every day. Try using a pedometer to keep track of every step in your Game Plan Food and Activity Tracker. A pedometer is a gadget that counts the number of steps you take. The number of steps in one mile depends on the length of your stride, but one mile equals roughly 2,000 steps. Each week, try to increase the number of steps you take by 1,000 (about 250 steps per day), aiming for a goal of 10,000 steps per day. If you decide to count steps as a part of your GAME PLAN, use this information to help you meet your 30 minutes of physical activity per day. Also, be sure to read the instructions for your pedometer.

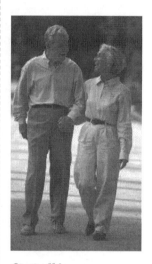

Start off by taking a 5-minute walk (or doing another physical activity that you like) on most days of the week.

Stretch it out.

Avoid stiff or sore muscles or joints by stretching after doing physical activity. Try not to bounce when you stretch. Perform slow movements and stretch only as far as you feel comfortable.

Make it social.

Try to schedule walking "dates" with friends or family members throughout the week. For family fun, play soccer, basketball, or tag with your children. Take a class at a local gym or recreation center. Organize a walking group with your neighbors or at work. When you involve others in your activities, you are more likely to stick to your program.

When you involve others in your activities, you are more likely to stick to your program.

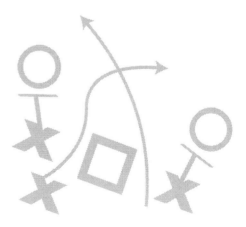

Have fun.

Getting more physical activity doesn't have to be boring. Turn up the music and boogey while cleaning the house. Go dancing with friends and family members. Play sports with your kids. Try swimming, biking, hiking, jogging, or any activity that you enjoy and gets you moving. Vary your physical activities so you won't get bored.

Keep at it.

Pay attention to small successes. The longer you keep at it, the better you'll feel. Making changes is never easy, but getting more physical activity is one small step toward a big reward—a healthier life.

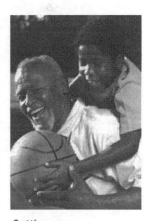

Getting more physical activity doesn't have to be boring.

Making changes is never easy, but getting more physical activity is one small step toward a big reward—a healthier life.

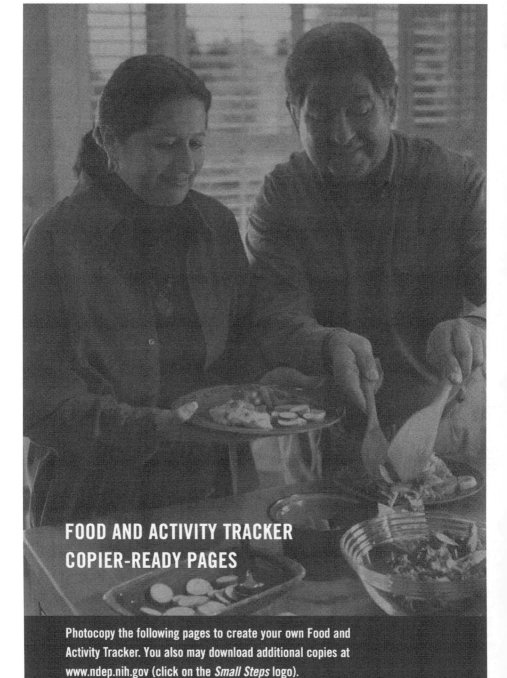

FOOD AND ACTIVITY TRACKER
COPIER-READY PAGES

Photocopy the following pages to create your own Food and Activity Tracker. You also may download additional copies at www.ndep.nih.gov (click on the *Small Steps* logo).

MY GAME PLAN
FOOD AND ACTIVITY TRACKER

NAME _____

DATE _____

FROM _____ TO _____

MY GAME PLAN THIS WEEK…

FOR CUTTING FAT GRAMS: _____

FOR CUTTING CALORIES: _____

FOR GETTING MORE
PHYSICAL ACTIVITY: _____

HHS' NDEP is jointly sponsored by NIH and CDC with the support of more than 200 partner organizations.

SAMPLE ENTRY:

DAY __Monday__   DATE __February 3__

DAILY FOOD AND DRINK TRACKER

TIME	AMOUNT/NAME/DESCRIPTION	FAT GRAMS	CALORIES
8:00 AM	1/2 cup oatmeal	1	73
	1 cup 2% milk	5	121

TO MAKE MORE WEEKLY TRACKERS: Make one (1) copy of this page. Place it on top of seven (7) copies of the next page. Trim the pages and staple in the upper left-hand corner. Fold to fit in your pocket or purse.

······ FOLD HERE ······

MY DAILY AND WEEKLY GOALS

	FAT GRAMS	CALORIES	MINUTES OF ACTIVITY
DAILY			
WEEKLY			

MY DAILY AND WEEKLY TOTALS

	FAT GRAMS	CALORIES	MINUTES OF ACTIVITY	WEIGHT
MONDAY				
TUESDAY				
WEDNESDAY				
THURSDAY				
FRIDAY				
SATURDAY				
SUNDAY				
WEEKLY TOTALS				POUNDS LOST

DAILY FOOD AND DRINK TRACKER

DAY	TIME	AMOUNT/NAME/DESCRIPTION	FAT GRAMS	CALORIES

MAKE SEVEN (7) COPIES OF THIS PAGE.

---- FOLD HERE ----

DAILY FOOD AND DRINK TRACKER (CONTINUED)

TIME	AMOUNT/NAME/DESCRIPTION	FAT GRAMS	CALORIES
TOTALS			

DAILY PHYSICAL ACTIVITY

TYPE OF ACTIVITY	MINUTES
TOTAL	

ADDITIONAL RESOURCES

National Diabetes Education Program
1-800-438-5383 or www.ndep.nih.gov and
click on the *Small Steps* logo

American Association of Diabetes Educators
1-800-TEAM-UP4 or www.aadenet.org

American Diabetes Association
1-800-DIABETES or www.diabetes.org

American Dietetic Association
1-800-877-1600 or www.eatright.org

Centers for Disease Control and Prevention
1-877-232-3422 or www.cdc.gov/diabetes

United States Department of Agriculture (USDA)
www.nutrition.gov

Healthier US Initiative
www.healthierus.gov

National Institute of Diabetes and Digestive and Kidney Diseases
National Diabetes Information Clearinghouse
1-800-860-8747 or www.niddk.nih.gov

Weight-Control Information Network
www.win.nih.gov/index.htm

National Heart, Lung, and Blood Institute
301-592-8573 or www.nhlbi.nih.gov

For on-line fat and calorie counters, visit these web sites:

National Heart, Lung, and Blood Institute
http://hp2010.nhlbihin.net/menuplanner/menu.cgi

United States Department of Agriculture
Nutrient Data Laboratory
www.nal.usda.gov/fnic/foodcomp/search/

Made in the USA
Middletown, DE
28 May 2021

40597971R00024